50 Sex Tokens For Your Pleasure :)

This Belongs To:

_____

Give me a lap dance in your own unique style...no one else turns me on like you do!

Good for a full body massage with a happy ending :)

Let me blindfold you and:

_____

_____

Undress slowly for me and let me masturbate just looking at you... you're so fucking hot!

Let me fuck you on/at/in

*Circle as desired

Role Play

Me:

You:

Good for one erotic movie of my choice.

You are my
sex slave
today

My 3 Rules Are:

1.
2.
3.

Good for sex position of my choice :)

*Fuck me! You're the best for giving me this! Don't ever think i don't know that.

Outdoor Sex

Anal.
Or if you (or i) are really not
into it ...
You suggest the dirtiest
alternative you can think of.
(Remember every little bit of
you turns me on...
I want nothing less!!!)

Ride me in a way to drive me crazy till i cum.

Spank me ☐
I want to spank you ☐

*tick as desired

*Circle depending on your mood

Let's fuck/make love
as we watch...

_____

Blindfold me and:

_____

_____

_____

_____

Cook me dinner naked
OR
Get naked, lay down on the kitchen table and put my fave desert all over you and let me eat it off slowly piece by piece...
You get to decide! See how considerate i am! :)

Shower Sex

No matter where we are or when, (i'll always look out for you and protect you)... let me fuck you when i give you this.

I want you to:

_____

_____

_____

_____

_____

Send me a really dirty text today...

Wear _____
for me and let's fuck
till i can't cum
anymore...

I want you to:

_____

_____

_____

_____

Let me _____
for however long i want,
listening to a soundtrack of
my choice.

Do that one
thing you know i
like but you
never want to do

I want you to:

_____

_____

Wear _____
for me and let's

_____

_____

I want you to:

_____

_____

Dress up for me wearing

_____

and let's go out to

_____

Sex Weekend Vacation or Staycation

* You & Me...Food, Drink and Sex All Weekend!

Made in the USA
Las Vegas, NV
21 February 2023

67883957R00057